Introduction

Back pain is a symptom

Backache is not an illness in itself, but a symptom. Its development means that something has gone wrong somewhere, although it may not always be clear exactly what.

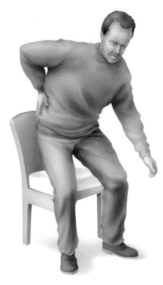

Most of us suffer from backache at some time or other. Usually it is an unpleasant, awkward but not desperately serious problem caused by some kind of mechanical stress or damage within the back which gets better fairly quickly. Poor posture, excessive stresses, and wear and tear problems may be at least partly responsible.

You should not be surprised that backache is so common when you realise that your spine is composed of many different structures, including bones, discs, ligaments, tendons, nerves, blood vessels and other tissues, all of which can be affected by mechanical damage resulting in backache.

In most cases the precise cause of the problem is not important. Backache is a symptom that will clear up; the purpose of treatment is to relieve pain and to make sure that you recover as soon as possible. Occasionally there may be a more severe underlying cause and detailed investigations are required to decide the right approach to treatment. Understanding how the back works will help us to protect our spines and recover more rapidly from attacks of backache.

This booklet aims to show you how the back works, what goes wrong, why back problems arise and how they are treated, and to give some indication of when further investigations and specialised help are necessary.

A growing problem

Backache is remarkably common. At any one time some 30 to 40 per cent of the population have backache and between 80 and 90 per cent experience it at some time in their lives. It affects both sexes and all ages from children to elderly people, but is most prevalent in the middle years.

ᴜerstanding
Back Pain

Professor Malcolm I.V. Jayson

Published by Family Doctor Publications Limited
in association with the British Medical Association

IMPORTANT

This book is intended not as a substitute for personal
medical advice but as a supplement to that advice for
the patient who wishes to understand more about his
or her condition.

Before taking any form of treatment
YOU SHOULD ALWAYS CONSULT YOUR MEDICAL
PRACTITIONER.

In particular (without limit) you should note that
advances in medical science occur rapidly and some
information about drugs and treatment contained in this
booklet may very soon be out of date.

© Family Doctor Publications 1997–2006
Updated 1999, 2000, 2001, 2003, 2004, 2005, 2006

Family Doctor Publications, PO Box 4664, Poole, Dorset BH15 1NN

ISBN: 1 903474 26 4

Contents

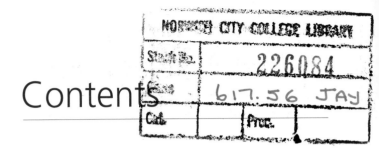

About the author

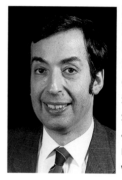

Malcolm I.V. Jayson MD, FRCP is Professor of Rheumatology and was Director at the Manchester and Salford Back Pain Centre. He has conducted extensive studies of the structure and function of the human spine, methods of measurement and trials of treatment, plus basic research on the mechanisms by which back pain develops.

What patients say

Back pain can take many forms, but the following complaints are typical:

'I work in a factory assembling components. By the end of the day I have a terrible aching pain low down in my back and I really don't know how much longer I can stand it.'

'I am not too bad during the day, but I wake up in the morning with a lot of pain and stiffness in my back, and I have to get up and move around before it eases.'

'I bent over to pick up a book from the floor and felt a sudden severe pain in the bottom of my back, and I couldn't straighten up.'

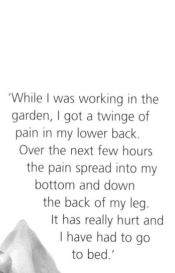

'While I was working in the garden, I got a twinge of pain in my lower back. Over the next few hours the pain spread into my bottom and down the back of my leg. It has really hurt and I have had to go to bed.'

Time off work

Backache is one of the most common reasons why people have to take time off work, especially in heavy manual industries. At particular risk are workers in the building industry and nurses who often have to undertake heavy lifts in awkward postures.

It's often hard to separate cause and effect: in other words, do the stresses in the job cause the backache, or is the person unable to do heavy work because he or she already has a bad back? In many cases, back pain follows some injury or a sudden twist. Much time is now spent training workers to avoid subjecting their backs to excessive stresses.

The scale of the problem

The amount of working time lost as a result of back problems has increased enormously in recent years. It is now running at some 100 million working days per year in England and Wales, two or three times more than 20 years ago. In fact, this dramatic rise does not mean that more people are being injured at work. Rather, it reflects the more concerned approach taken by both workers and employers to the effects of back pain. The result is a dramatic escalation in the costs of back pain to our society. This is now calculated as nearly £6,000,000,000 (six billion pounds) per year for the medical treatment provided, the benefits received and loss of production – a phenomenal sum.

The increase in the numbers of people disabled by back problems has led to a complete rethink of our approach to back pain and how it is treated. In this booklet I provide the most up-to-date views based on the latest research on the treatment of back pain, and explain how we are attempting to reduce the frequency and severity of this problem.

KEY POINTS

- Backache is a symptom not a disease

- Acute episodes of back pain, although unpleasant, usually get better quickly

- Backache affects 80–90 per cent of the population at some time in their lives

How the spine works

The vertebral column

The spine or backbone is known medically as the vertebral column. Its role is to support the whole body, be capable of bending and twisting in all directions, and at the same time protect the vital structures such as nerves that run through it. What's more, it has to last a lifetime. No engineering structure comes anywhere near meeting such specifications, so it is hardly surprising that problems can arise from time to time.

Vertebrae

The human spine consists of a column of bony blocks known as vertebrae, which sit one on top of another, joined together by tough ligaments to form the vertebral column.

There are seven cervical vertebrae in the neck, twelve dorsal or thoracic vertebrae in the upper and middle back, and five lumbar vertebrae in the lower part of the spine. The fifth lumbar vertebra is known

The versatility of the spine

The spine or backbone is a truly amazing engineering structure, allowing a huge range of movement while supporting the body and the vital structures, such as nerves, that run within it.

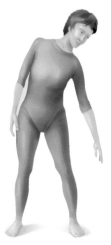

The spine can bend sideways

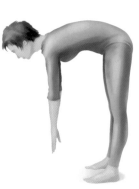

The spine can bend forwards

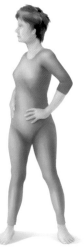

The spine can twist

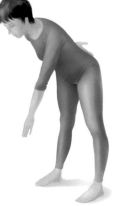

The spine can bend and twist at the same time

as L5 and sits on the sacrum, which in turn is connected to the coccyx – the tail bone. The sacrum consists of several vertebrae that have joined together. The sacrum is joined at its edges to the pelvis – the ring of bone that carries the trunk and which in turn is supported by the hips.

Discs

The spine is not a rigid structure. It is able to bend and twist because there are flexible cushions or discs between each of the vertebrae. Each disc is a flat, biscuit-shaped structure with a jelly-like centre called the nucleus and an extremely strong outer skin called the annulus.

Facet joints

The vertebrae are also joined to each other by pairs of small joints which lie at the back of the spine, one on either side. They can be affected by strain or by wear and tear and may develop bony swellings, causing pressure on nerves.

Nerve network

The nervous system resembles a telephone network carrying messages from your brain to various parts of your body and back again. Messages that pass down the nerves make muscles contract and so control movements such as walking. Those travelling up the nerves carry sensations which eventually reach your brain so that you experience sensations such as touch and pain.

The spinal cord and nerves

A 'cable' of nervous tissue, known as the spinal cord, extends from the brain down the spine inside the canal

The spine – side view

Viewed from the side the human spine has a definite curve.
The spine is not a rigid structure; it is able to bend and flex
because there are cushions or discs between each of the
vertebrae. The vertebrae attach to the skull at the top and
the pelvis at the bottom.

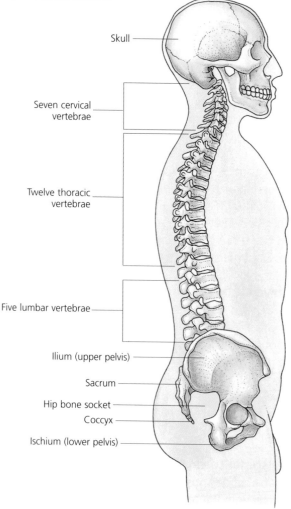

Skull

Seven cervical
vertebrae

Twelve thoracic
vertebrae

Five lumbar vertebrae

Ilium (upper pelvis)

Sacrum

Hip bone socket

Coccyx

Ischium (lower pelvis)

The spine – back view

Viewed from the rear the human spine consists of a vertical column of bony blocks called vertebrae, which sit one on top of another. The vertebrae are numbered in descending order according to their location:

- Seven cervical vertebrae = C1–C7
- Twelve thoracic vertebrae = T1–T12
- Five lumbar vertebrae = L1–L5

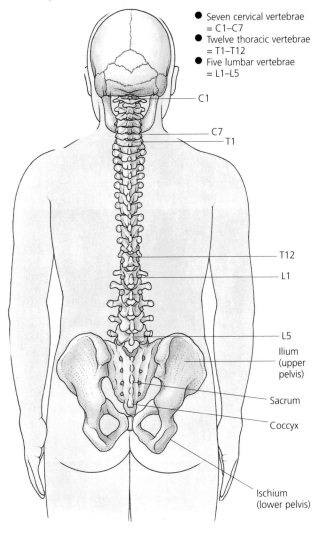

C1

C7
T1

T12

L1

L5

Ilium (upper pelvis)

Sacrum

Coccyx

Ischium (lower pelvis)

The structure of the spine

The vertebrae are separated from one another by flexible intervertebral discs. Each disc is a flat, biscuit-shaped structure with a jelly-like centre (nucleus) and an extremely strong outer skin (annulus).

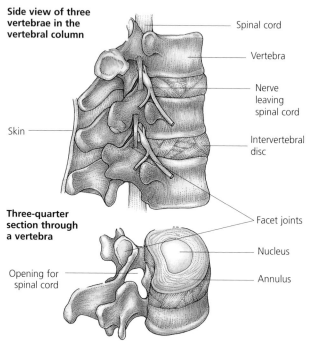

Side view of three vertebrae in the vertebral column

Spinal cord

Vertebra

Nerve leaving spinal cord

Skin

Intervertebral disc

Three-quarter section through a vertebra

Facet joints

Nucleus

Opening for spinal cord

Annulus

formed by the vertebrae. The nerve roots separate from the spinal cord, run for short distances within the canal itself and emerge in pairs, one on each side, from the sides of the vertebral column to supply the body, the arms and the legs.

What happens in back injuries

The fact that the spinal cord carries messages to and from the body means that, if it is damaged, the 'connection' may be affected, which can lead to the

The nerve network

A cable of nervous tissue, known as the spinal cord, connects the nerves of the limbs and torso to the brain. The spinal cord runs through a protective canal within the bony vertebral column. Nerve roots emerge in pairs from the sides of the vertebrae.

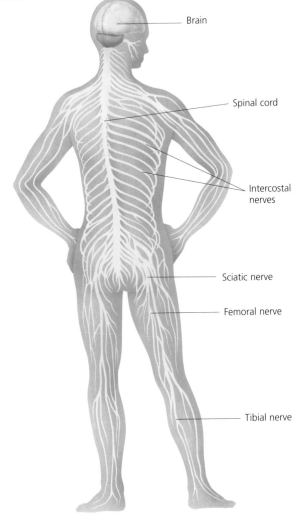

Brain

Spinal cord

Intercostal nerves

Sciatic nerve

Femoral nerve

Tibial nerve

loss or alteration of sensation, development of pain and weakness of movements. This is what happens when people become paralysed after a serious accident.

The number of limbs paralysed, that is whether the affected person can move the arms and not the legs, or whether all four limbs are paralysed, depends on where the spinal cord has been damaged.

If the injury is in the neck, paralysis and loss of sensation can affect both the arms and the legs. However, if the injury is in the thoracic or lumbar segments – below arm level – then only the leg muscles are affected. Fortunately most back problems damage only the nerves and not usually the spinal cord.

Pain can develop in the back itself, resulting from direct injuries to ligaments, tendons, joints and other structures. As the same nerves that supply these tissues in the back also supply the legs, patients may feel the pain as though it were arising from the legs.

In addition, there may be pressure directly on the nerves, producing pain, alteration in the sense of feeling and weakness in the legs.

Investigating back pain

It is clear that the back is a very complicated structure. When there has been some injury, back pain can arise for several different reasons. Very careful analysis would be necessary to determine what has happened in any individual. Fortunately, most acute episodes of back pain get better without the need for specific forms of intervention.

As a result very detailed tests to determine the particular injuries causing problems are generally not required. However, when symptoms are more serious and prolonged, it becomes important to determine exactly what is going wrong. Very careful examination and diagnostic tests, including some of the newer forms of computer imaging, may then become necessary.

KEY POINTS

- The vertebral column consists of vertebrae joined by discs and facet joints. The disc has a jelly-like central nucleus and an extremely strong outer skin, the annulus

- Pain may arise from damage to a wide variety of structures

- The pain is transmitted by the nerves. The ways that these are stimulated are complex and depend upon the particular tissue or type of nerve that has been affected

- As most acute episodes of back pain get better quickly, usually there is no need for very detailed tests to determine the precise cause

What is pain and what can we do about it?

What is pain?

Pain is a sensation that we all feel yet find extremely difficult to describe. Putting into words the unpleasantness of the experience is no easy task.

Much thought has gone into the description of pain and pain experts agree that pain is 'an unpleasant sensory and emotional experience with actual or potential tissue damage or described in terms of such damage'.

There is an emphasis on the emotional response that exacerbates how we feel pain. Some people may describe discomfort but put up with it, yet others with a similar injury become extremely distressed. Our emotional responses to the pain lie at the heart of understanding the pain experience, particularly in chronic (long-lasting) pain situations.

Modern pain management is aimed at:

- relieving the tissue damage that may cause the pain

- blocking the pain pathways

- helping us to cope with painful situations so that the patient can get on with everyday life despite ongoing symptoms.

In general pain is a warning that something is going wrong. It is ringing an alarm bell to tell us to protect against or relieve some form of injury.

Categorising pain

Pain can arise as a result of various causes:

Cause of pain	Example
• Injury to tissues	• Cut or graze to skin
• Inflammation	• Joint pain in arthritis
• Injury to nerves	• Trapped nerve in vertebral column

Where does the pain lie?

If you injure your back and develop backache, you identify the pain as arising in the back, but actually our appreciation of it is in the brain. Without the brain there is no pain.

It follows that treatment may be directed not only at the injured area but also at how our nervous system handles the pain message.

A memory of pain

Sometimes the actual injury heals but the brain and central nervous system have a memory of the pain so that the patient continues to believe that the back is still painful, and indeed it is painful but the problem lies with this memory of the painful experience. This is real pain. It is not imagined but the mechanism for producing the pain sensation lies within the nervous system rather than in the back itself.

This memory for pain develops particularly in people with chronic back problems. In those with long-lasting symptoms, increasingly the central nervous system is generating this painful experience and amplifying the severity of symptoms that are arising from the back.

As a result treatment of back pain will depend on the development and stage of the problem.

Treatment of back pain
Acute and sudden onset of back pain

In the acute stage with pain of sudden onset or relapsing episodes, it primarily arises as a result of the damage in the back and pressure on nerve roots, and treatment is directed accordingly with perhaps a short period of rest, followed by active mobilisation with physiotherapy, osteopathy and chiropractic as necessary. Relief of pain may be with simple painkillers or sometimes anti-inflammatory drugs (see page 79).

Chronic back pain

In chronic persistent backache, careful investigation is necessary to ensure that there is no other underlying problem. Additional means of treatment will include medicines that calm down the central nervous system, reducing the excitability of nerve fibres in the brain's spinal cord that are generating the painful sensation.

Rehabilitation and pain management programmes become important and may include cognitive–behavioural therapy (CBT) which helps chronic back sufferers understand the nature of their problem, and learn ways of coping with it and how to live a normal life.

With this understanding of how we feel pain we can move forward to look at common back problems and what to do about them.

KEY POINTS

- Pain is an unpleasant experience that suggests to the patient actual or believed tissue damage

- Pain may arise as a result of local injury and inflammation or of injuries to nerves

- Although backache seems to arise in the back, the actual feeling process is in the brain

- There is a memory of pain within the nervous system so that sensation of pain can persist after the tissue injury has healed

- Emotional responses can add to the distress caused by pain

- There are different treatment strategies for acute backache and chronic long-lasting back problems

Some common back problems

Now we know the make-up of the spine, it is easier to understand where and why problems can arise.

Non-specific back pain

Many people who have trouble with their backs experience brief episodes of pain from which they make a full recovery. No firm diagnosis is made and so their back pain is called non-specific. Detailed investigations are not necessary and often it is not possible to identify the particular underlying cause. Sometimes the person has tender areas over the spine or between the sacrum and the iliac bone of the pelvis. The pain may be caused by strains of ligaments, tendons or other soft tissues.

Although the cause is usually uncertain, terms that imply that your doctor has actually made a diagnosis – such as lumbosacral strain and sacroiliac strain – are often used. The term 'non-specific back pain' is preferable because it does not suggest that we know the cause of your particular problem. Further investigation to pinpoint the cause is necessary only if the back pain fails to settle.

Discs – slipped or burst?

Most people have heard of a 'slipped disc' but it is a rather inaccurate name because discs actually cannot slip. They can wear, split or burst. What happens is that, after some stress on the spine – often involving bending, twisting or lifting – the disc bursts or prolapses and the jelly-like central nucleus is squeezed out through a split in the outer annulus.

Effects of a prolapsed vertebral disc

Under stress the intervertebral disc can rupture, forcing out the nucleus which may then press on and aggravate the spinal nerve root. This pain can often be felt down the leg, sometimes as far as the foot.

Cross-section through prolapsed intervertebral disc

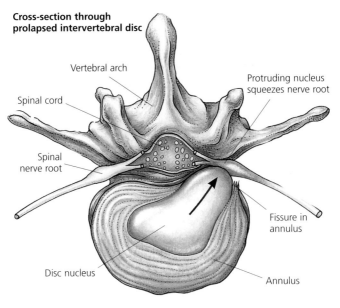

Vertebral arch

Protruding nucleus squeezes nerve root

Spinal cord

Spinal nerve root

Fissure in annulus

Disc nucleus

Annulus

We now believe that most discs that prolapse in this way previously had some wear-and-tear changes and the stress on the spine triggered the problem. In other words, the disc was already abnormal and would have burst sooner or later anyway. The particular stress probably just acted as a 'final straw'.

The jelly-like material, having been squeezed out, presses on the nerve running next to the disc, causing severe pain in the back that spreads down the leg and sometimes as far as the foot. You may feel numbness and tingling, particularly in your lower leg and foot. Some of your muscles may become weak and the ankle jerk reflex, tested by tapping your Achilles' tendon with a tendon hammer, may be lost. The site of these changes helps the doctor to identify exactly which nerve has been damaged.

The pain caused by a burst disc can be very severe. Usually the symptoms will slowly get better and eventually disappear completely. However, once the disc has burst, it is permanently weak and there is always the risk of a further bout of back pain.

Sciatica

As the greatest weight and bending forces are experienced in the lower part of the lumbar spine, the nerves most often damaged are the fifth lumbar nerve root (which leaves the spine between the fourth and fifth lumbar vertebrae) and the first sacral root (which leaves the spine between the fifth lumbar vertebra and the first part of the sacrum). These two nerves join together to form the sciatic nerve which runs down the back of the leg to the foot. Pain arising because of damage to this nerve is known as sciatica.

The lumbar region of the spine

The greatest weight and bending forces are experienced in the lower part (lumbar region) of the spine. The nerves most often damaged are the fifth lumbar nerve root (between L4 and L5) and the first sacral root (between L5 and S1).

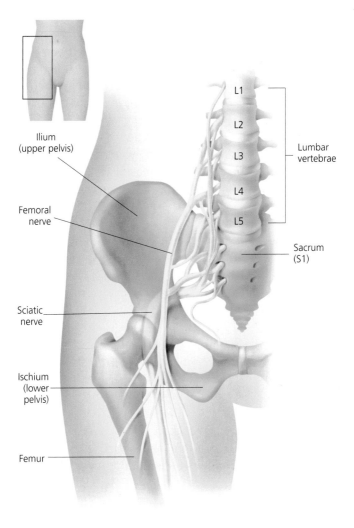

Ilium
(upper pelvis)

Femoral
nerve

Sciatic
nerve

Ischium
(lower
pelvis)

Femur

L1

L2

L3

L4

L5

Lumbar
vertebrae

Sacrum
(S1)

Sciatic nerves

The sciatic nerves are the largest nerves in the body. This diagram shows a burst of the L5/S1 disc pressing on the nerve root of the sciatic nerve and causing pain that may be felt as leg pain.

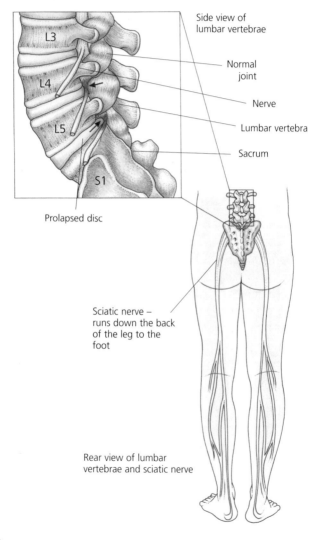

Side view of lumbar vertebrae

L3

L4

L5

S1

Normal joint

Nerve

Lumbar vertebra

Sacrum

Prolapsed disc

Sciatic nerve – runs down the back of the leg to the foot

Rear view of lumbar vertebrae and sciatic nerve

Wear and tear – spondylosis

Spondylosis, or wear and tear of the spine, is very common. Indeed these changes start at about the age of 25 and are present in almost all of us by the time we are middle-aged. This is one of the main reasons why athletes are at the peak of their performance in their early twenties.

The lower back bears the weight of your whole body as well as anything that you're carrying, and does most of the bending and twisting. This is why wear-and-tear changes of the spine are most common in the lumbar region, and are called lumbar spondylosis.

Lumbar spondylosis is most likely to occur at the lower levels, particularly between the fourth and fifth lumbar vertebrae (L4/L5) and the fifth lumbar vertebra and the first segment of the sacrum (L5/S1), and leads to sciatica (see page 22). It affects both the discs and the facet joints.

Some material is lost from the disc and from the cartilage or gristle lining the facet joints. The bone at the margins of the discs and facet joints enlarges, making movement more limited and so stiffening the spine. It may press on nerves, ligaments and other structures, causing pain.

However, this is not as depressing as it sounds. The fact that you have these wear-and-tear changes does not mean that you are bound to get backache. Many people have quite severe wear-and-tear changes with few or no problems, whereas others with relatively minor changes suffer incapacitating bouts of pain. Wear-and-tear changes of this sort are generally of only minor significance.

How wear and tear affect the spine

Lumbar spondylosis (wear and tear in the lower part of the back) is extremely common. Here the bone at the margin of the intervertebral disc and facet joint has enlarged, pressing on the nerve root and causing pain.

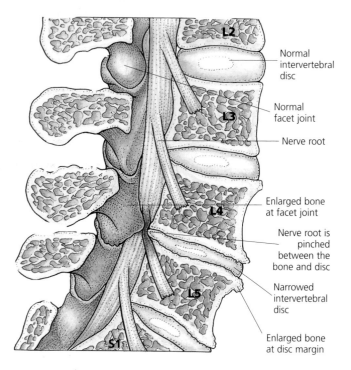

Normal intervertebral disc

Normal facet joint

Nerve root

Enlarged bone at facet joint

Nerve root is pinched between the bone and disc

Narrowed intervertebral disc

Enlarged bone at disc margin

Lumbago

One of the most common back problems is recurrent spells of acute pain which may spread to the buttocks or one of the thighs. While the attack lasts, your back may feel stiff and tender as well. When the symptoms are very severe the condition is called lumbago. The pain can last a day or two or up to a couple of weeks each time. Sometimes it then disappears completely or it may persist or recur. The symptoms are made worse by poor posture and heavy lifting.

X-rays frequently show the presence of lumbar spondylosis, but surveys have revealed that these changes are often found in people who don't have any symptoms. It is therefore difficult to assess the part they have played in causing pain. As a result of this, the term 'non-specific back pain' is often used to describe lumbago.

Nerve problems

Nerves easily get squashed within the vertebral canal and as they emerge from the sides of the vertebral column by damaged discs, facet joints or vertebrae. When a nerve is squashed its ability to pass messages is affected. When this happens, you may experience pain or a sensation of numbness or tingling in the area supplied by the nerve, and the muscles it controls in your leg or foot may become weak. The spinal cord transmits these sensations to the brain – it is a bit like interference on a telephone wire, producing unpleasant noises and poor quality sound. In fact, current research indicates that it is a lot more complicated than that. Changes within the spinal cord itself can affect the pain message. This may explain why some patients continue to experience widespread and prolonged symptoms when the original nerve damage has healed and there is little evidence of much wrong with the back.

Coccydynia

This is the name given to pain at the tail end of the spine or the coccyx. Usually no cause is found. A soft cushion ring may be used to make sitting more

Trapped and squashed nerves

Nerves can easily become squashed within the vertebral canal and as they emerge from the vertebrae. When a nerve is squashed you may feel pain, tingling and numbness, and experience muscle weakness in the area that the nerve supplies.

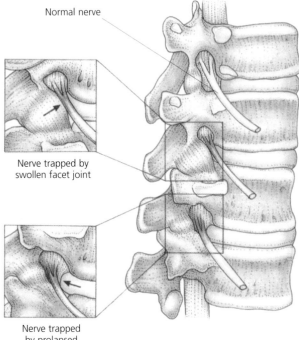

Normal nerve

Nerve trapped by swollen facet joint

Nerve trapped by prolapsed intervertebral disc

comfortable, but the condition usually settles by itself with time.

Neck problems

This section deals only briefly with common neck disorders. The neck shares the same basic structure as the rest of the spine, and is therefore also prone to disc problems and wear-and-tear changes.

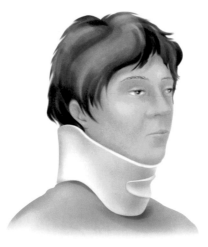

Neck collar.

While pain in the lower back commonly shoots down the legs, neck pain may involve the shoulders and arms. For uncomplicated neck problems, treatment with rest, painkillers and perhaps physiotherapy usually suffices. A padded neck collar is helpful to ensure that the neck is properly supported and rested.

Acute stiff neck syndrome

Many people have had the experience of waking up with a stiff and painful neck, often it seems for no particular reason. Movement may be possible only in one direction and the muscles of the lower neck may be tender. There are no other problems with the rest of the back or the arms or legs. The pain is associated with muscle spasm and will settle with a neck collar and painkillers in three to four days. Occasionally very gentle neck traction (applying a steady pulling force) may help.

Whiplash

This is common after a car accident, when the sudden impact gives no time for muscles to brace, and the head moves like a pendulum on the neck. In the simplest cases only ligaments in the neck are sprained, and the pain and stiffness that result are caused by the neck muscles going into spasm as a protective mechanism. If there are no other problems, painkillers, a short period of rest, return to physical activity and sometimes physiotherapy are all that are required. In some cases pain persists for longer than six weeks, and it may be that the initial injury was more serious, causing damage to the discs or other structures, and has led to nerves being damaged or trapped. More detailed investigation is needed. Treatment may involve surgery. When pain remains severe for several months, it becomes more likely that there will be continuing disability.

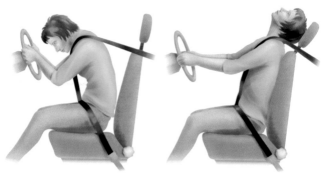

Sudden deceleration
as occurs when hitting
a vehicle in front

Sudden acceleration
as occurs when your car is
hit from behind

Whiplash injury to the neck in a motor vehicle accident.

Disc problems in the neck

Discs can also prolapse in the neck, although this is less common than in the lower back. The neck is extremely stiff, and pain may shoot down one arm. Strength, sensation and reflexes in the arm may be lost. In the majority of cases, the pain will settle with rest, pain relief, traction if necessary, and then a period of gentle activation with a collar. Physiotherapy to strengthen the neck muscles is also useful.

Wear-and-tear problems

These changes are extremely common in the neck, and are known as cervical spondylosis. They may cause no problems at all, or lead to neck pain with headache and/or arm pain. Neck movements are reduced, and some patients have a tender spot in the trapezius muscle which lies between the neck and the shoulders. Again, the arms may become weak and lose their reflexes. There may be tingling or pins and needles in the arms.

In the most serious cases, the distorted bone and ligaments can press on the spinal cord, affecting control of the arms and legs or an artery in the region, called the vertebral artery. This leads to dizziness, a buzzing in the ear and pain behind the eyes.

Many people who have cervical spondylosis also have low back pain. The principles of treatment are the same: rest in a collar, physiotherapy, anti-inflammatory drugs and pain relief. Surgery may be necessary for a small proportion of patients.

KEY POINTS

■ Discs do not slip but they can burst

■ Sciatica is caused by damage to either of the two nerves that join to form the sciatic nerve running down the lower limb

■ Wear and tear or spondylosis of the spine is very common as you get older, but does not inevitably lead to back pain

■ Neck problems have many similarities to back pain

Treating back pain – the first steps

Finding the cause of the problem

Most of us get sudden episodes of pain in the back from time to time, usually lasting only a day or so. Apart from being careful you don't need to do anything about it and it is soon forgotten. Some people, however, may develop more severe attacks of pain which limit their activity and their ability to work.

Despite all our modern technology, in many cases we are not able to determine the exact source of the problem. It could well be the result of some damage to the ligaments, muscles or other soft tissues, but often your doctor may be unable to determine the precise cause. The good news, however, is that generally it does not matter because most of these acute attacks of back pain will get better rapidly.

The most common problem is simple backache in which the pain is confined to the back or may spread into the buttock or upper thigh. Sometimes it may extend right down the leg, affecting the sciatic nerve and giving rise to sciatica (see page 22). Pressure on this nerve may come from a damaged disc or other structures, causing pain and sometimes numbness and tingling running down your leg. Sciatica suggests that there has been some nerve damage and that recovery is likely to be slow.

Severe symptoms

Occasionally, a person may develop more severe symptoms which means that they need to be seen quickly by a specialist. This will be necessary for anyone who experiences any problems controlling the bladder or bowel, any numbness in the groin or rectal area, or severe leg weakness, because it could be a sign of more severe nerve damage.

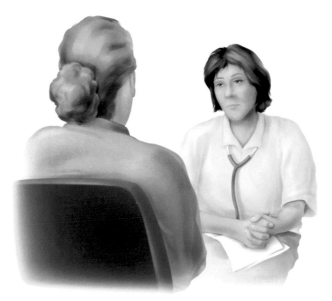

Details of the complaint are all important.

Assessing the problem

Usually, when you have an acute back problem, the person treating you will ask for details about how and when the pain started and what has happened since, and give you a physical examination. Questions you may be asked include:

- Is the pain in one area or is it more general?

- Does the pain shoot or spread anywhere, for example, the leg?

- How did it come on – suddenly or gradually? If gradually, over what period of time?

- Was the onset associated with any activity?

- Does anything make the pain worse?

- What is the pain like first thing in the morning?

- Are you otherwise well? Have you lost weight/got a cough/other problems?

A pain that started on lifting a heavy object is sharp and limited to a small area, and is easier with rest, is likely to be uncomplicated and should get better rapidly.

However, if the pain began gradually over many months, does not seem to be linked to movement and is becoming more severe, and there are other problems such as weight loss, the cause may be more serious and special investigations may be necessary.

You may be sent for an X-ray, but usually this is not necessary. Although it may well show that you have some wear-and-tear changes, these features are common in people without backache and so don't have much influence on the choice of treatment. Each X-ray exposes you to radiation, which is why they

When examining your back, the doctor may:

- Look for signs of curvature, and observe the way that it bends and how you walk.

- Feel your back for tender spots or areas.

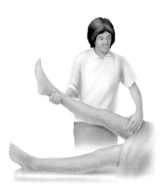

Examining the back.

- Perform the straight leg-raising test. The doctor lifts each leg straight up, when you are lying flat on your back. If there is a problem with the sciatic nerve, this will bring on the pain.

The straight leg-raising test.

- Perform the femoral stretch test. The doctor places you lying on your front, then slowly bends each knee in turn. If there is a problem with another nerve called the femoral nerve, this will bring on the pain.

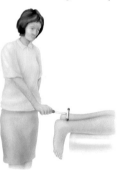

The femoral stretch test.

- Look for loss of sensation or weakness in the legs.
- Check your reflexes.

Testing the ankle reflex.

should be reserved for people with severe back pain that has not responded to simple treatment and for those who have more complicated back problems.

You are unlikely to need more detailed types of imaging such as computed tomography (CT) or magnetic resonance imaging (MRI) scans (see pages 69–70)

Treatment
Simple remedies
For most people with acute backache, only very simple treatment is needed:

- Simple pain-relieving tablets such as paracetamol or ibuprofen. These tablets have few side effects and are usually all you'll need. You can ask your doctor for stronger painkillers, which are available on prescription, if you feel that you need them.

- A short period of bedrest can be helpful for people in severe pain, but too much can actually aggravate the problems. If you're in severe pain, you should rest lying flat in bed for at most a couple of days. After that, you should start to move around again, taking care to protect your back, but aiming to return towards normal physical activity as soon as possible.

- A cold pack – such as a bag of ice or frozen peas – against your back helps in some people to relieve the pain. In others heat in the form of a heating pad or a hot shower is comforting. However, neither is likely to make any long-term difference.

For most people, simple remedies such as these are enough and the pain will usually clear within a few days or a couple of weeks. You should aim to get back to normal physical activity as soon as possible. It is important that you take note of the advice in the chapter on how to protect your back in order to reduce your chances of having another attack in the future (see page 43).

Seeing a therapist

You may, however, be one of the unlucky ones whose pain does not disappear completely. If you still have a problem after about four to six weeks, you need to see a therapist. This might be:

- a doctor with special expertise in the appropriate treatment techniques
- a physiotherapist
- an osteopath
- a chiropractor.

Physiotherapy

Physiotherapy is the more traditional form of physical therapy, and usually involves the use of heat, gentle massage and exercise to help someone regain movement, strength and suppleness. Many physiotherapists are also trained in manipulation.

Osteopathy and chiropractic

Osteopathy and chiropractic tend to concentrate on joint manipulation. In general, a chiropractor may use quick, gentle, specific thrusts, whereas an osteopath uses slower, more general movements. All therapists will give advice on the care and protection of the back.

In practice, however, it is doubtful whether there is much to choose between these techniques, because the principles behind treatment are the same, including

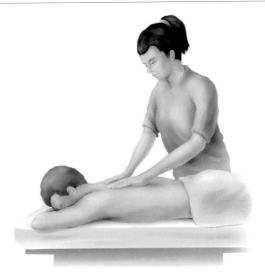

Physiotherapy is the more traditional form of physical therapy and usually involves the use of heat, gentle massage and exercise to regain movement.

physical activation of the affected area with various types of exercise and manipulation.

Surgery
Treatment for sciatica also involves pain-relieving tablets, rest and remobilisation, but progress is often a lot slower. Sometimes people with this particular problem have to be referred for surgery to relieve the pressure on the nerve. More information on persistent back pain is given in the next two chapters.

Recurrent back pain
The usual pattern of most acute back episodes is recovery, commonly in a few days but sometimes taking a week or even a few weeks. People with a history of backache are likely to develop further

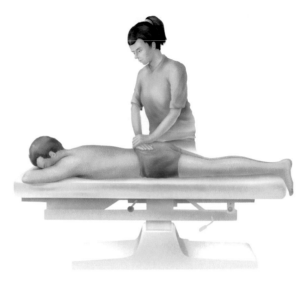

Osteopathy and chiropractic tend to concentrate on joint manipulation.

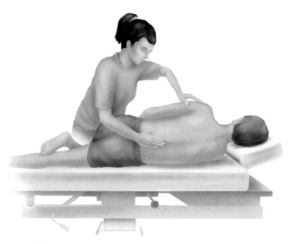

Manipulation of the joints of the spine can help to restore mobility and alleviate pain.

episodes in the future. Sometimes future back pain occurs as a result of an accident or an exceptional load, but for many people acute relapses may be precipitated by quite trivial physical activities. Understanding how the back works and minimising stresses on the spine, together with improvement in physical fitness, will help to prevent further recurrences of back pain.

KEY POINTS

- Most acute back pain is simple backache.

- A small proportion of people have sciatica and a few have more complicated problems

- Simple backache usually responds to pain relief, a short period of bed rest if necessary, and early physical activation and return to work

- If your condition fails to improve, you may need to see a therapist or a specialist who may undertake further investigations and treatment

Protecting your back

Minimise back stress

Some people who start off with an underlying back weakness go through repeated bouts of back pain, often because of a combination of poor posture and excessive stresses. We now know how different positions and loads affect the back and may lead to back problems, but you can teach yourself how to minimise the stresses you place on your back. These lessons are actually important for all of us, but especially for anyone who gets back pain and would like to try to prevent further attacks.

Improve your posture

How we stand and sit is important and may greatly affect our ability to cope with back pain. Taking care over this will minimise a lot of stresses on your spine. Standing badly can stretch the spinal ligaments and cause aching and stiffness in your back. The following tips will help improve your posture:

- Standing incorrectly will eventually lead to back pain. Stand upright with your head facing forwards, your back straight and avoid slouching. Stand with your weight evenly balanced on both feet, legs straight and your body upright with the natural curve of your spine

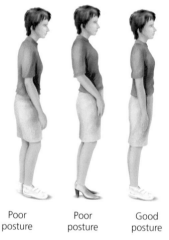

Poor posture   Poor posture   Good posture

- Keeping still in one position for a long time particularly in low soft armchairs is an important cause of aching and stiffness.

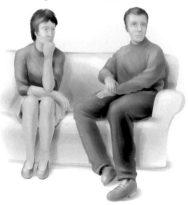

- When sitting at a desk, ensure that you can sit upright with a support in the small of your back. The desk should be of sufficient height and with sufficient leg space so that you are close enough to sit upright and work comfortably. There should be enough room beneath the work surface so that you can get close to your work without having to bend forwards, and also to allow free movement of your legs and feet.

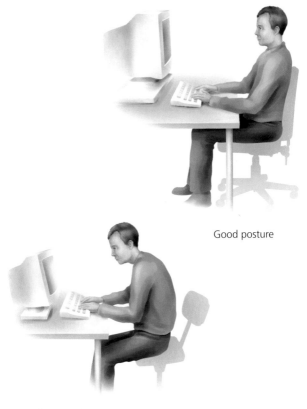

Good posture

Poor posture

- When you're working at a bench check that it is high enough so that you can stand upright with a good comfortable working posture.

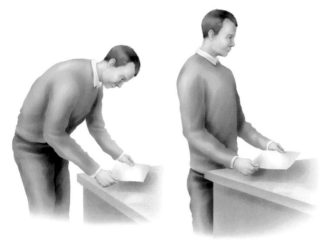

Poor posture   Good posture

Examine your shoes

Women who get back pain should not wear high heels. Such shoes tip the lower part of your body forwards, and you then arch your upper body backwards to compensate, so putting stress on your back. Also it's better to opt for shoes that don't have hard leather soles because they send shock waves up through your skeleton as your heels strike the ground, and often aggravate back problems.

Cushioned soles and heels or shock-absorbing insoles can reduce this and often make walking much easier. I recommend trainers because they are so comfortable and minimise these sudden shock waves.

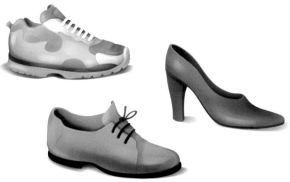

Choose your shoes carefully

Sitting correctly

Many chairs are poorly designed. Often the worst are
low armchairs and easy chairs that look temptingly soft
but hold your back in a rounded position, causing
severe aching and stiffness. Perching on a stool with
your back bent forwards often aggravates backache
and stiffness, so avoid it if you can. You will be most
comfortable in an upright chair which supports your
lower back, maintaining the normal slightly backward
curve of the lumbar part of your spine. If necessary,
you can make your own lumbar support using a small
cushion or a rolled-up towel, or put a back rest or
lumbar roll behind the small of your back.

Comfort in your car

Backache is common in all of us who spend long
periods driving. Anyone who is prone to backache can
experience particular problems. In recent years, car
manufacturers have paid much more attention to the
design of the car seat and to the driving position in
order to minimise backache. However, we still find
seats that are poorly designed, holding the back in a

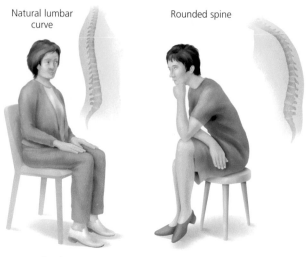

Natural lumbar curve

Rounded spine

Good posture

Poor posture

Try to sit upright with the natural curve of your spine maintained and both feet flat on the floor. You will be most comfortable in an upright chair that supports your lower back.

rounded position. Sitting for a long time in this posture can cause excruciating back pain. The best car seats have a built-in adjustable lumbar support, and the height, seat and back angles can be altered to suit the individual driver. The foot controls should be squarely in front of your feet and not at an angle because this causes constant spine twisting. Adequate wing mirrors will help you avoid having to twist round, and power steering will lessen the strain on your spine when manoeuvring at low speeds.

Lifting correctly

Many back problems develop during lifting. Frequently this arises when load bearing is combined with bending forwards, and maybe also with a twist on the

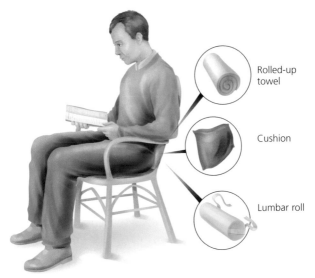

Rolled-up towel

Cushion

Lumbar roll

If necessary you can make your own lumbar support using a small cushion or a rolled-up towel. Back rests and lumbar rolls can also be bought.

spine. There are some simple practical guidelines that help to protect the back and reduce the risk of back trouble.

Is the object too heavy?

The first priority when lifting is to decide whether the load is too heavy or bulky to move on your own. There are no hard and fast rules about the maximum weight that can be lifted safely. Much depends on the circumstances, the size, shape and weight of the object, and where it has to be moved to, and on your personal physical strength and health.

The strain on your spine is much greater if the object is held at arm's length rather than close to your body. Someone with back problems can carry much less weight and bulk than a healthy adult. On the whole men can carry heavier loads than women and young people.

The object should be held close to your body and not at arm's length. Get a firm grip with the palms of your hands and the roots of your fingers and thumbs, rather than with your fingers alone. Heavy objects should not be lifted above shoulder level as this produces tremendous strain on the spine. The same principles apply when putting things down as when picking them up: with one foot in front of the other and at right angles to it, hold the object close to your body, and then crouch down so that the knees spread apart and set the object down between your feet.

Monitor your movements

Bending forward and twisting movements combined with carrying a heavy load are the most likely to stress your spine and produce back problems. Avoiding this type of stress is important for all of us, but especially for anyone with a back problem.

Your sleeping posture

A lot of people get backache in bed. This is often because they have a poor quality mattress and base that sag under the weight of their body. Most of us sleep on our sides so sagging produces a sideways bend in the back that may lead to considerable aching and stiffness. You can largely stop this happening by sleeping on a bed that does not sag so easily. The ideal bed is one with a firm, well-sprung mattress and base, although it does not need to be hard.

In fact, it may be a mistake to buy a very firm hard bed in the belief that it is good for your back because

How to lift objects from the floor (kinetic method)

Lifting objects from the floor is the origin of many back problems. Bending forwards places great strain on the ligaments of your back and is a common cause of acute spine pain.

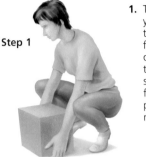

Step 1

1. The right way to lift is to place your feet apart, at right angles to each other, and with the front foot pointing in the direction to which the object is to be moved. This puts you in a stable position and prevents you from twisting your back in the process of lifting and then moving off.

2. Crouch down, bending your hips and knees but keeping your back straight. Your whole spine may be inclined forwards but it is important to avoid bending your back. In this position, your knees are well apart and the object is positioned between them and kept close to your body. You can get a good, firm grip and the lift is performed using your leg muscles.

Step 2

Step 3

3. Once you are upright, you should carry the load close to your body without twisting your back. Put it down carefully, using the same procedure in reverse. This is known as the kinetic method of lifting. Many industries train their workers to use this technique automatically, but it should be the lifting method used by everybody.

it can be so uncomfortable that you don't sleep well. When you're choosing a bed, spend some time lying on it to ensure that it is firm but comfortable.

Unfortunately, a well-sprung, quality bed can be very expensive. An alternative, if you have an overly soft mattress, that is almost as effective is to place a firm board on top of the base and underneath the mattress. It should run the full length of the bed and be thick enough not to bend under the weight of your body. Three-quarter-inch (two-centimetre) block board seems a very good choice for this purpose.

Too many pillows

Your whole spine should lie as straight as possible so that neither your spine nor your neck bends sideways during the night. Too many pillows put a sideways twist on your neck that will be transmitted down your back. It is usually better to use only one pillow so that your head and neck are in line with the rest of your body when lying on your side.

Stay in shape

If you are overweight, you are putting additional strain on your back, and this may mean you have a poor posture. Losing weight becomes important not only for your back, but also because it is good for your general health.

Exercise

Physical fitness and exercise form an important part of prevention and treatment if you are prone to back problems. We believe that exercises help to prevent back pain by increasing the ability of the trunk to cope with loads. There are many different types of exercise,

Your sleeping posture

Many people get backache in bed. Often this is because they have the wrong mattress for their body weight and size.

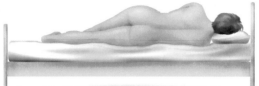

Correct posture – the mattress is firm enough to support the body while absorbing the impression of the body (e.g. buttocks and shoulders), so keeping the spine straight.

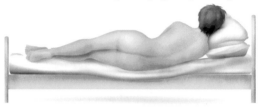

Poor posture – the mattress is too soft and the spine is curved. Too many pillows cause excessive spine curvature.

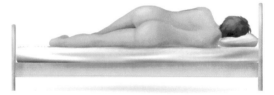

Poor posture – the mattress is too firm. All of the body lies on the mattress, distorting the naturally straight spine.

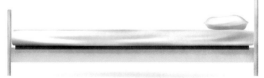

A well-sprung bed can be expensive. An alternative that may be effective is to place a firm board under the full length of the mattress.

such as aerobics, weight-training, stretching and bending exercises (see pages 74–7). Most important is keeping fit and strengthening your spine muscles.

Some exercises can make back pain worse. If you have a back problem, it is important to be careful and to concentrate on the exercises designed for strengthening the back and stomach muscles, rather than those aimed at forcing back movements.

Back care in the home

Careful planning will minimise stresses on the spine and help to protect the back. Avoid having to bend and lift heavy saucepans from cupboards or the oven. If you do have to handle them, apply the principles of safe lifting.

Avoid sitting in low armchairs. An upright seat that is high enough for you and a back rest to preserve the normal hollow in the back will be a lot more comfortable. Avoid bending over the sink. A shower may be a lot easier than getting in and out of the bath. Housework does not all have to be done in one go. Pace yourself and spread out the work over several days. Avoid heavy vacuum cleaners, particularly if they have to be carried up and down stairs.

Back care in the office

Poor working conditions aggravate back complaints. Although there are well-established principles, it is remarkable how many office workers have to put up with poorly designed working conditions. It is important not to spend prolonged periods working in one position. There should be frequent breaks and I normally recommend that five minutes in every hour be spent away from the keyboard undertaking some other type of physical activity. This might be filing, sorting papers or making a cup of coffee.

A good chair will be stable on a swivel base and adjustable in height. The seat back has an adjustable tilt and is also shaped to preserve the lumbar curve. The seat may be tilted very slightly forward, but the height should be such that feet rest flat on the ground or on a footrest. They should not dangle because this causes pressure on the thighs.

The desk should be large enough to accommodate work comfortably. Ideally it will be adjustable in height so that you can work with the elbows at 90 degrees.

The computer screen should be positioned so that the top of the screen is at about eye level. There should be space on the desk or on a keyboard rest so that the wrists can be rested when not typing.

A sloping writing surface can also be a lot more comfortable.

Attention to these details helps to make it a lot easier for the back sufferer to cope with office life.

KEY POINTS

- Good posture is important for preventing backache

- The shoes that we wear and the chairs that we sit on can also affect our backs: avoid sagging chairs and high heels

- When lifting an object, follow the 'kinetic method of lifting' and avoid lifting very heavy objects

- Make sure that your bed has a good, firm but comfortable mattress and avoid use of too many pillows.

What causes persistent back pain?

Identify the cause of back pain

Some people suffer persistent or chronic back pain, and need careful investigation to find out why. Once the cause is identified, a proper treatment programme can be planned.

By far the most common cause of chronic back pain is some mechanical disorder in the back. However, in a small proportion of people, pain is the result of inflammatory diseases, disorders of bone, tumours or problems in the abdomen or pelvis.

Chronic mechanical back pain

Many people suffer persistent pain in the back which may spread into the buttock or the leg. Often, the pain is aggravated by physical activity and by certain postures. The spine is a very complicated structure and many different things can go wrong. The following are common causes of chronic mechanical back pain.

Lumbar spondylosis or ageing changes

X-rays of the back frequently show signs of ageing changes in the intervertebral discs and facet joints. Indeed they are present in almost every older person. Although people with these ageing changes more often get backache than those without, there is only a poor correlation with the presence of symptoms. It is possible for a person to have quite severe X-ray evidence of wear and tear, and yet be symptom free. For this reason signs of wear and tear in the spine should be treated with caution. Just because you have them and also have backache does not mean that the changes are the cause of the symptoms. Nor does it mean that someone who has these changes but no backache is bound to develop back problems or become disabled in the future.

In lumbar spondylosis, the pain is felt across the low back, sometimes worse on one side than the other. The pain is worse with physical exercise and bending, and made easier by rest. However, some people tend to stiffen when lying in one position. This may be particularly noticeable first thing in the morning or after prolonged sitting in an easy chair. The pain can spread into one or other buttock and sometimes into the back of the thigh.

On examination back movements are usually limited, but often this is only on certain types of movements, whereas other movements are relatively free.

Prolapsed or burst intervertebral disc

Under stress the disc may burst – usually backwards and to one side – so that it presses on a nerve, leading to pain in the back, spreading down the leg. Commonly the disc was already showing marked evidence of wear-and-tear damage and was seriously weakened. The particular stress precipitated the development of the burst that was about to occur anyway. When the disc prolapses, the person may develop sciatica (see page 22). The problem may persist and lead to long-term pain and disability.

The person will describe pain in the buttock usually spreading down the back or the outside of the thigh to the back of the calf and sometimes into the foot, usually the top or outer aspect. Frequently, it is accompanied by tingling or pins and needles, known technically as paraesthesiae. These can be very painful and also there may be the sensation of numbness.

The examination reveals evidence that the nerve is trapped. When the leg is kept straight and lifted upwards there is a lot of pain and the movement is limited. There may be weakness of certain movements of the foot and the ankle reflex can be lost. There may be a reduction in the ability to feel in the area of the damaged nerve.

Hypermobility or very flexible joints and backache

Some people have remarkably flexible joints. They can bend forwards with the legs straight to place the palms of their hands flat on the ground. The joints of the arms and legs can bend to a remarkable degree. This is known as hypermobility. Many sportsmen and sportswomen, trapeze artistes and professional dancers are hypermobile because this facility enables them to undertake physical activities far beyond most of us.

Paradoxically, in later years hypermobility predisposes to development of joint symptoms. It is likely that repeated excessive movements have led to the development of wear-and-tear changes and

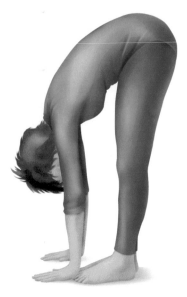

Hypermobility.

overstretching of ligaments. In particular it is an important cause of back problems. It is remarkable how well back movements are preserved in these patients, and sometimes they have difficulties in convincing their doctors that there is anything wrong because their movements appear to be so good.

Inherited variations in the spine

We are all different shapes and sizes and our spines vary accordingly. Some people are born with an extra lumbar vertebra or one too few or with abnormally shaped vertebrae. These variations are usually unimportant and do not cause their owners any pain.

Spondylolisthesis

Sometimes one vertebra slips forwards on top of the one below because of a weakness in the supporting arches of the vertebral column. This is called a 'spondylolisthesis' and can cause pain because it results in over-stretching of nerves or ligaments.

This slipping may be the result of failure of the supporting bones in the back of the spine to develop properly or of wear-and-tear change between vertebrae.

Spinal stenosis

The nerve roots run down from the spinal cord within the column of vertebrae and then emerge from the sides of the spine through narrow openings (each known as a foramen, several as foramina). They then run down into the legs.

We all have spinal canals and foramina of different sizes and shapes. Some are smaller than others so that nerves that run through them are at particular risk of getting squashed.

When the narrowing affects the central canal of the vertebral column, it is known as central spinal stenosis and may lead to pain, numbness and tingling in the legs, which develop on walking and are relieved by rest. These symptoms are quite similar to the leg problems associated with a poor blood supply to the legs. The pain is also made worse by arching backwards and relieved by bending forwards.

When the narrowing affects the foramina through which the nerve roots emerge, patients may develop persistent unremitting pain of the sciatica type. This is known as foraminal stenosis. Surgery to relieve these types of nerve pressure can be very effective.

Fibromyalgia

People with this condition develop a range of symptoms. They experience widespread pain across the back, spreading up the back of the chest into the neck and the limbs. They often have tender points, particularly over the sacroiliac joints, the shoulder blades, and the inside and outside of the elbows and knees, but also elsewhere. Frequently, these people have had a variety of detailed tests, but no particular abnormality can be pinpointed. Many people with fibromyalgia are very upset and depressed; they feel tired and lacking in energy. It is often difficult for doctors to decide whether the persistent pain has led to the depression or whether the depression has led them to feel pain more severely.

It may well be that the explanation lies in changes in the way pain sensations are transmitted in the spinal cord.

Many people with this condition sleep poorly and wake up in the mornings feeling unrefreshed, with generalised aches and pains and stiffness. Some research suggests that this poor sleep rhythm may be responsible for the problem. People with fibromyalgia often have other problems such as irritable bowel syndrome and migraine.

Other causes of back pain

Although most backache is the result of mechanical disorders such as those I have described, in a small proportion of people it is a symptom of some other illness. For this reason you should always be thoroughly assessed by a doctor, particularly when back pain develops for the first time or when its nature suddenly changes. Other causes of back pain include the following.

Infection

Fortunately this is uncommon, but occasionally people with severe back problems are found to have chronic infection in the discs or elsewhere.

Ankylosing spondylitis

This is an inflammatory form of arthritis in which the effects are concentrated on the back. Sometimes it can attack the joints of the arms and legs, and occasionally other body tissues.

Most often it starts in young adults, usually men. However, women sometimes get it and it can start at any age. The initial problems appear in the joints between the sacrum and the pelvis (sacroiliac joints) and may then spread up the spine. As it advances, it can cause stiffening of the back with a pronounced stoop and in severe cases the spine may end up completely rigid.

In contrast with people who have mechanical backache, those with ankylosing spondylitis usually find that their pain and stiffness are aggravated by rest and relieved by exercise. They often toss and turn in bed and wake up in the early hours of the morning with aching and stiffness. Many get up in the night and do some physical exercise in order to obtain relief. As the condition becomes more severe, the aching and stiffness may last longer throughout the day.

Your doctor will examine you and probably organise blood tests and X-rays to confirm the diagnosis.

Bone disorders

The skeleton provides the scaffolding that supports the soft tissues of the body. Unlike a metal framework, bone is a living material in which the constituents are constantly being renewed. There are several types of disease that lead to weakening and deformity of the bone and may make you more prone to fractures.

Osteoporosis

This is a common form of bone disease. Most often it affects women after the menopause when hormonal changes lead to weakening of the bone structure, although men can and do get it too. Some people develop osteoporosis as a result of hormonal disorders such as Cushing's disease or as a complication of treatment with certain steroid drugs.

When the bone is weakened, tiny fractures occur very easily and the vertebrae become squashed. Some people

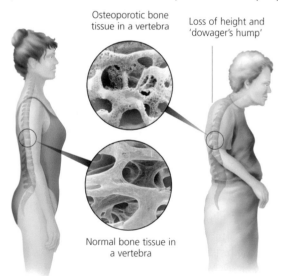

Osteoporotic bone tissue in a vertebra

Loss of height and 'dowager's hump'

Normal bone tissue in a vertebra

Osteoporosis is a common form of bone disease mainly affecting women after the menopause. Hormonal changes lead to a thinning of the interior structure of the bones, making them weaker and more prone to fracture. Weakened vertebrae may become crushed, causing loss of height and severe bending forwards.

experience repeated attacks of severe back pain as a result and gradually develop a stoop. The loss of height and severe bending forwards, which often affect older women, are usually caused by osteoporosis.

Osteomalacia

People with this condition lack calcium and vitamin D, which can be the result of a poor diet low in dairy products, failure to absorb calcium from the bowel or lack of sunlight.

Their bones become weaker, so that they are more prone to fractures and pain.

Paget's disease

This condition causes the bone suddenly to start growing very quickly; it affects elderly people. The new bone is abnormal and soft and may fracture easily or press on nerves and ligaments, causing pain.

Tumours

Occasionally back pain may be caused by a tumour developing in the back or spreading from elsewhere. Although it is a rare cause of backache, the possibility has to be ruled out, which is why it is important to have a proper medical assessment.

Referred pain

This is the term doctors use to describe pain that you feel in your back, but that actually has its origin somewhere else in your body.

Not all back pain is caused by problems in and around the spine – for example, it might be caused by disorders in the abdomen or pelvis. Stomach ulcers, gynaecological problems and some other conditions can result in pressure on nerves, causing back pain. When there is some link between bouts of pain and a woman's periods, doctors will consider whether there may be a gynaecological cause. Sometimes it is not obvious that the problem is actually arising in the abdomen or pelvis.

KEY POINTS

- There are a number of medical conditions that cause back pain, including many mechanical disorders

- Back pain can also be a symptom of some other illness, such as inflammation, infection, bone disorders, referred pain, etc.

- Changes associated with the ageing process can cause back problems in elderly people

- In women after the menopause, osteoporosis can cause back pain and bending of the spine

Treating persistent back pain

First step – getting a diagnosis
Your medical history

For your doctor, the most important part of assessing your back problem is finding out from you exactly how the pain started and what has happened since, together with other medical features. You will then have a physical examination. That may well be all that is necessary.

Blood tests

As we have seen, most backaches have a mechanical cause, so the results of blood tests are normal. However, such tests are useful when investigating possible inflammatory and other causes of back pain. In particular, ankylosing spondylitis (see page 63) is associated with the presence of a certain white blood cell type known as HLA-B27. If this is not present when your blood test results come back, you are very unlikely to have this condition. However, a blood test

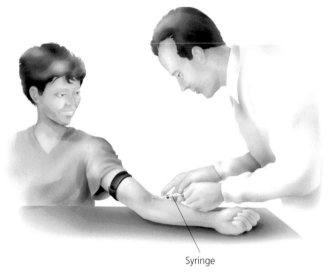

Syringe

Taking blood for testing.

result that shows the presence of HLA-B27 does not prove that you have ankylosing spondylitis, because this white cell type is also found in about eight per cent of people who do not have this condition.

X-rays

Vast numbers of spine X-rays are taken but the majority are unnecessary. The only people who really need them are those with severe back pain that has failed to get better with simple treatment and those with complicated problems. Unnecessary X-rays should be avoided as each involves some, albeit slight, exposure to radiation.

Radiculography

When we look at X-rays of the spine we are actually studying shadows of the bones. This means that we

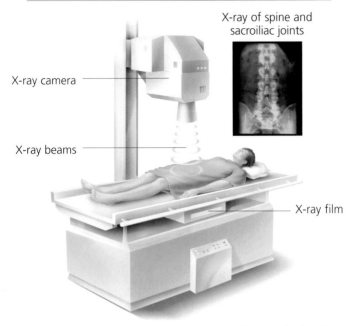

X-ray of spine and
sacroiliac joints

X-ray camera

X-ray beams

X-ray film

Spine X-rays are usually reserved for those with severe back pain
and complicated problems.

cannot see the soft tissues such as the nerves and discs
within the spine. In a radiculogram (myelogram), dye
that is opaque to X-rays is injected into the spinal
column. When a disc has burst, the column of dye will
be indented so that the exact location of the damaged
disc can be identified on the X-ray.

CT scans

CT stands for computed tomography. CT scans enable
doctors to use X-rays to obtain a clearer view of the
internal structures of the vertebral column. In particular
the inner outlines of the bony structures can be
examined and some details of the discs can be seen.

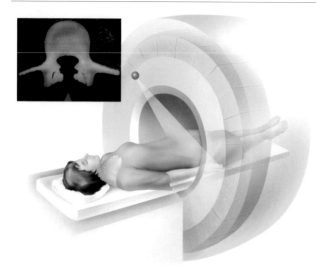

Computed tomography (CT) is much more sensitive to changes in tissue density than an X-ray. An X-ray tube and detector rotate continuously around the patient as the patient is moved through the gantry. The CT scan shows a a series of cross-sections through the body, creating a 'map' of the region being studied.

MRI scans

MRI stands for magnetic resonance imaging and is the latest scanning technique. It involves the use of very strong magnetic fields rather than X-rays, and is particularly good for studying the nerves, ligaments and discs within the bony structures. Having an MRI scan may be a very claustrophobic experience and some people have difficulty tolerating it. Relaxants are often used. In some centres an open MRI machine is available for very distressed patients

CT and MRI scans are now widely available. However, it's not always clear who can really benefit from such scans. As with X-rays of the back, the changes that they reveal often correlate poorly with symptoms.

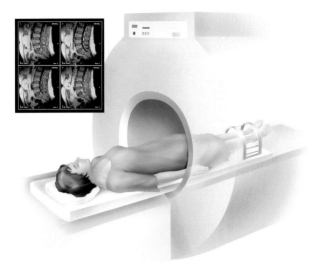

Magnetic resonance imaging (MRI) allows the soft tissues of the body (e.g. lungs and brain) to be visualised. The MRI scanner uses magnetic waves to disturb the nuclei of hydrogen atoms in the tissues of the body. The tissues of the body emit signals which are then measured in a strong magnetic field, forming a picture that doctors can interpret.

Non-drug treatment for back pain

How chronic back pain is treated depends on whether it is caused by mechanical problems – the most common kind – or by some other disorder.

Caring for your back

Physical activity is good for people with chronic back problems. You should try to keep active and to exercise, although you do need to take some sensible precautions. You have to be careful, for example, to avoid over-stressing your back and to be aware of your posture when standing, sitting and lifting. Lifting heavy loads is not a job for you.

Physiotherapy

Views on treatment have changed dramatically in the last few years. We now believe the principal role of the physiotherapist is to get you mobile again and restore you to normal levels of activity as soon as possible. It is important that you be referred to a physiotherapist if your back problem has lasted more than a few weeks and is in danger of becoming chronic.

The physiotherapist will teach you how your back works, what can go wrong and how to protect the back against excessive stresses, and teach you exercises aimed at restoring your mobility so that you can start to function normally again.

The exercise programme will normally be tailored to your individual needs, but will include ones to strengthen your back and abdominal muscles, together with pelvic tilt exercises.

Sometimes, the physiotherapist will apply various forms of heat such as an infrared lamp or short-wave diathermy, or other treatments such as ice packs or cooling aerosol sprays, ultrasound or massage. Such treatments do not cure the long-term problem but can be extremely soothing and relaxing. Their special value is often as a preliminary to other forms of treatment such as exercises, which otherwise would be very painful.

Traction, like many of the treatments of back pain, has been used since ancient times. You lie on a special traction table with one harness around your lower chest and another around your pelvis; the two halves of your body are then gently pulled apart. The idea is to stretch damaged joints and relieve pressure on damaged nerves. It helps at the time, but its long-term value is doubtful and its use is becoming restricted. It is not worth rushing out to buy any of the expensive gadgets available on the market for home traction.

Exercises

There are many different types of exercise for people with chronic back pain, and the choice depends very much on the nature of your particular problem. Some exercises may help one type of backache but make another worse, so be careful when planning your own exercise programme.

You should discuss exercises first with your physiotherapist. The various types of exercise include those already described, aimed at strengthening the back and abdominal muscles (known as isometric exercises), and those that improve movements of the back. It is important to avoid any exercises that make the pain suddenly worse. It is better to undertake a specific amount of exercise which is gradually increased each day.

For more severe chronic back problems, and in particular for people who have become disabled, exercises are often undertaken in a special heated pool. This is known as hydrotherapy. The exercise programme is performed under the supervision of a physiotherapist. This does seem a very pleasant and helpful method of promoting recovery for those with more severe back pain.

Sport

Sportsmen and -women should keep active and return to sport as soon as possible after a bout of severe pain. The safest options are walking, swimming and cycling. Contact sports such as rugby are risky because sudden, unexpected and forceful movements of the back can undo several weeks of gradual improvement.

Exercises that may help relieve chronic back pain

A simple and safe programme of exercises should be undertaken in a graduated and gradually increasing fashion. Initially do the following exercises once or twice daily and then gradually increase up to six times each day as your back allows.

For many people, other types of exercise are required, but these should be performed only under the guidance of a physiotherapist because certain exercises can make some patients worse. Much depends on the particular problems in each individual case.

1 Lie flat on your back on the floor. Keep the legs straight and lift each heel in turn, just off the floor. Repeat.

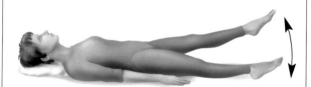

2 Lie flat on your back on the floor with a pillow under your head. Fold your arms. Lift your head and shoulders just off the floor and then lie flat and relax. Repeat.

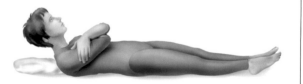

If any of these exercises aggravate the back pain, then they should not be performed.

3 Lie flat on your back on the floor. Tense your stomach muscles and flatten the small of your back onto the floor, then relax. Repeat.

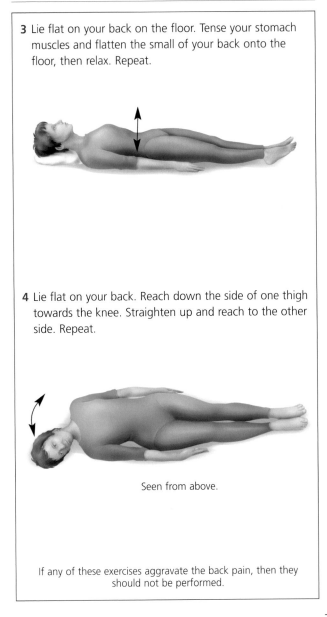

4 Lie flat on your back. Reach down the side of one thigh towards the knee. Straighten up and reach to the other side. Repeat.

Seen from above.

If any of these exercises aggravate the back pain, then they should not be performed.

5 Lie flat on your back on the floor. Bend your knees so that your feet are flat on the ground, then lift your bottom in the air by tightening the stomach muscles, keeping the back straight. Repeat.

6 Lie on your stomach on the floor, then do press-ups with your hands, but keeping your back straight. Repeat.

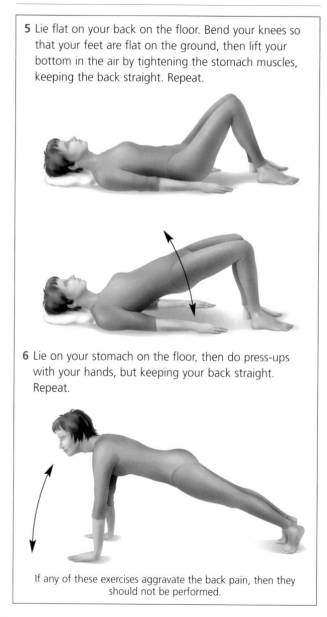

If any of these exercises aggravate the back pain, then they should not be performed.

7 Kneel on all fours. Arch and hollow your back. Then flatten your back. Repeat.

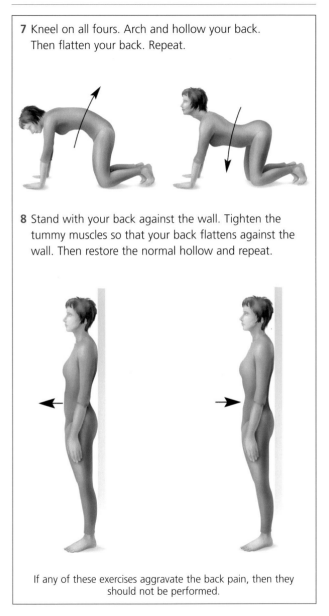

8 Stand with your back against the wall. Tighten the tummy muscles so that your back flattens against the wall. Then restore the normal hollow and repeat.

If any of these exercises aggravate the back pain, then they should not be performed.

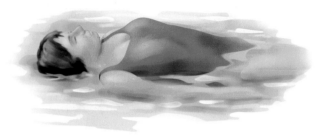

Swimming is one of the safest forms of exercise for back problems. Swim on your tummy or on your back, whichever is most comfortable.

Mobilisation and manipulation

If back pain is caused by mechanical displacement of one of the joints or discs, then it should be possible to put things right by manipulation of the spine. This is the theory underlying the various techniques of mobilisation and manipulation. There is wide variety in the techniques practised by physiotherapists, osteopaths, chiropractors, physicians and orthopaedic surgeons.

Some manipulators apply forces directly to the vertebrae in the spine whereas others use the shoulders and pelvis as levers. There is no agreement on the problems for which manipulation is useful, when the different types of manipulation should be used and the relative usefulness of these treatments by the various practitioners. Manipulation can hasten your recovery from an acute episode of back pain but it is doubtful whether it provides real benefit for chronic back pain.

In general manipulation appears to be safe, although a few people find that it makes their back problems worse. There is a very small risk of nerve damage when manipulation is performed under anaesthetic.

Medicines and tablets to relieve back pain

The main purpose of drugs is to relieve pain. The two main types used are pure pain relievers known as analgesics and those – known as anti-inflammatory drugs – that also control inflammation in the area of damage. The character of the back problem is often helpful in indicating which type of drug will be most effective.

Painkillers

Paracetamol is the most commonly used painkiller. You can take up to six or eight 500 milligram tablets a day and it is very safe provided you don't exceed this dose. You can buy paracetamol by itself or combined with other drugs such as codeine from chemists without a doctor's prescription.

There are several stronger analgesics such as dextropropoxyphene and dihydrocodeine which are often combined with paracetamol, but these are available only on prescription.

Anti-inflammatory drugs

You'll find these particularly helpful if you have a lot of stiffness in bed and when you wake up in the morning. Their main role is to reduce inflammation, but they are effective painkillers as well. Aspirin was the first anti-inflammatory drug but it can cause indigestion and abdominal upsets, and larger doses may give you ringing noises in your ears and interfere with your hearing. Ibuprofen is available over the counter in pharmacies and seems to produce far fewer problems.

There are alternative anti-inflammatory drugs available on prescription, such as naproxen, diclofenac, piroxicam, ketoprofen and many others. These are generally taken in tablet form. A lot of research has gone into producing newer versions that need only be taken once or twice a day rather than every few hours – an obvious advantage.

All the anti-inflammatory drugs can cause abdominal upsets, so you may be prescribed an anti-ulcer treatment to take at the same time. Sometimes the anti-ulcer treatment is combined with the anti-inflammatory drug in a single tablet or capsule. We now know that the anti-inflammatory effects of these tablets are caused by blocking the COX-2 (COX is cyclo-oxygenase) enzymes and the indigestion effects are caused by blocking the COX-1 enzymes.

The coxib story

Efforts have been made to develop new anti-inflammatory drugs that do not cause indigestion and stomach upsets. These are known as coxibs because they are targeted at the COX-2 enzymes, which are the inflammatory enzymes that cause pain, and do not block COX-1, which is an enzyme that protects the stomach. They seemed to be helpful. Unfortunately the first of these was rofecoxib (Vioxx), which, we now know, has a serious adverse effect of carrying an increased risk of heart attacks and strokes. In consequence rofecoxib and certain other coxibs have been withdrawn.

Celecoxib (Celebrex) seems to carry less risk than rofecoxib and is still available. There is, however, continued study of its risks and benefits.

There is also a small risk of skin reactions, which can be severe with coxib drugs.

The current advice is that coxibs such as celecoxib must not be used in patients with ischaemic heart disease, or those who have angina or heart attacks, cerebrovascular disease such as a stroke or with poor blood circulation in the legs.

Caution is also indicated in those with risk factors for cardiovascular problems such as high blood pressure, a high cholesterol level, diabetes and smoking.

Decisions about whether to use drugs such as celecoxib depend upon a careful assessment of the medical indications and risk factors, and they should be used in the lowest effective dose and for the shortest period of time.

In general pure painkillers are preferable to anti-inflammatory drugs but in some patients provide insufficient relief. An anti-inflammatory drug may prove the answer but should be taken only after discussion with your doctor. An anti-ulcer treatment taken at the same time either separately or combined in one capsule may prevent abdominal upset.

Muscle relaxants

If you are one of those people who develop quite severe spasm of the back muscles, which is very painful, you may find that muscle relaxant tablets are a help.

Anti-epileptic drugs

Neuralgic pains are sudden electric shock sensations shooting from the back down the leg, often accompanied by painful tingling and numbness. These symptoms seem to result from over-sensitivity of the damaged nerves.

People with epilepsy have over-sensitive brain cells which fire off in an uncontrolled way, causing them to have seizures (or fits). The drugs used to counter that problem can also be effective in relieving neuralgic pain.

Tricyclic antidepressants

Some people who have chronic back problems develop widespread pain and often their skin becomes hyper-sensitive so that it is tender to even light pressure. Alteration in the pain-processing system in the central nervous system probably underlies this. This type of pain is not helped by conventional pain-relieving tablets. There may be similar biochemical changes in the central nervous systems of people who are clinically depressed, and the drugs used for treating depression, such as amitriptyline, can be effective for treating this kind of pain.

Rubs, creams and gels

Rubbing a pain-relieving cream or gel into the back is sometimes very helpful. Part of the benefit comes from the various medications in the rub, but also the massage itself seems to help.

There are three types of rubs which act in different ways. One type may suit you rather than another. It is well worth trying the different types of rub before giving up the process.

Salicylates

Simple rubs contain a small amount of salicylates and other medicines and cause an increase of blood supply and a sense of warmth, together with pain relief. Examples include Movelat, Transvasin, etc. They may be applied two or three times a day if they help.

Anti-inflammatory

The anti-inflammatory medicines taken by mouth are also available as creams and gels. They penetrate the skin and relieve pain in the local area. Only a small amount gets into the general circulation. There are several different types of cream, all available over the counter. These include ibuprofen, diclofenac, ketoprofen and others, and appear under various trade or proprietary names, such as Oruvail Cream, Voltarol Emulgel, Traxam Cream, etc.

Capsaicin

More recently, there has been special interest in an extract from chilli peppers known as capsaicin. This has the effect of releasing the pain-producing substance from nerve endings. When initially applied, it often causes a burning sensation of the skin, but when used two or three times a day, after a couple of days this settles down and is followed by pain relief when the nerves are completely depleted of the pain-producing substance.

Some patients use this preparation only intermittently, with the result that they only get the burning and do not experience the pain relief. They can discard this type of treatment as useless. It is important to use it two or three times a day and to persist with it in order to get the benefit. Examples include Axsain and Zacin creams.

Injections

Injections can be very helpful for certain types of back pain. They take a number of different forms depending on the precise nature of the problem.

For tender spots

Some people with back problems have one or two very localised tender areas in their back – perhaps in the superficial tissues, the ligaments connecting the vertebrae, the sacroiliac joints or elsewhere. Your doctor can identify the painful areas by feeling your back carefully while you are lying flat in a relaxed position. The tender spots may then be treated with an injection of a small amount of local anaesthetic and a powerful steroid, such as cortisone. Steroids also have long-lasting anti-inflammatory action. After the injection, you will usually be free of pain for two to three hours as a result of the anaesthetic, but then the pain may return for 24 hours or so. However, after that period, some people find that their pain diminishes dramatically. How long this relief lasts varies considerably from one person to another, but for many it is long lasting. Cortisone used in this way does not cause the adverse effects that may develop when it is taken regularly by mouth.

Facet joint injections

Sometimes the problem arises in the facet joints at the back of the spine, and this can also be treated by means of an injection using a fine needle. It is usually done under X-ray guidance so that the injection can be positioned in precisely the right place in the joint.

Epidural injections

An epidural injection is given into the spine around the linings surrounding the spinal cord and nerve roots. A local anaesthetic with a small amount of a cortisone-like drug is injected. You may be offered this if you have sciatica that has improved after a severe attack but has not cleared up completely.

Other treatments
Acupuncture

Back pain can be very difficult to control. Sometimes, the symptoms are relieved by blocking the passage of nerve impulses up the spine to the brain.

Acupuncture was first developed in China between 2,000 and 3,000 years ago. It was thought to work by altering the balance between the two opposing life forces known as yin and yang. Acupuncture is often used in Western medicine today. We now know that it stimulates the release of natural chemicals known as endorphins and enkephalins within the brain and spinal cord, which can block the passage of the pain sensations.

Sterile needles are inserted into the skin and then rotated to produce stimulation. Some acupuncturists

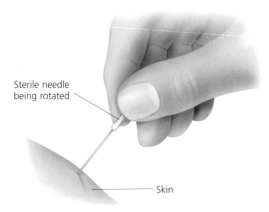

Sterile needle being rotated

Skin

Acupuncture is a method of pain relief that involves insertion of fine sterile needles into specific points on the body. The needles are then rotated to produce stimulation. Acupuncture does not work on everybody.

use the traditional Chinese acupuncture sites but for many this is out of custom rather than belief.

Acupuncture does not work on everybody. Some people respond well, others derive only short-term benefit and need repeated treatment, and for some acupuncture makes no difference at all.

Transcutaneous electrical nerve stimulation (TENS)

The problem with acupuncture is that inserting needles into the skin and applying stimulation is a highly skilled technique and you have to attend a special clinic to have it done. TENS, on the other hand, is a treatment

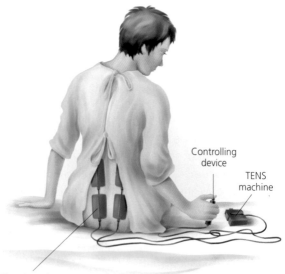

Controlling device

TENS machine

Electric pads

Transcutaneous electrical nerve stimulation (TENS) involves fixing electric pads to the skin of your back. Tiny pulses of electricity stimulate your skin, acting in a similar way to acupuncture.

that you can give yourself in your own home. You fix electric pads coated with a special electrical conducting jelly to the skin of your back. These are then connected to a battery and stimulator which you wear on your belt.

When you switch the gadget on, multiple tiny pulses of electricity stimulate your skin, and you can adjust the strength, frequency and length of time of each impulse to suit yourself. The electrical stimulation feels like a tiny pricking sensation in your skin. It acts in a similar way to acupuncture by stimulating nerves, and releasing substances in the brain and spinal cord that block the sensation of back pain.

This technique is useful for someone with chronic back pain who can switch on the stimulator whenever he or she needs it. TENS does not help everybody but can be remarkably successful for some.

Corsets

The lumbar support or corset consists of a firm body belt stretching from the rib cage to the pelvis, with strengtheners behind which may be flat steel strips moulded to the shape of the back. Wearing a corset limits your back movements and increases the pressure within your abdomen, and so it may relieve back pain. Unfortunately, wearing a corset for a long time can lead to permanent back stiffness and in the long run many corsets do as much harm as good. We now believe that, for most people, the aim should be to restore movements to the back as soon as possible, which is why corsets are now used only rarely.

Surgery

It is estimated that only about one operation is needed for every 2,000 attacks of back pain. Surgery should be considered only if:

- your symptoms have not responded to other treatment
- you have severe and persisting pain
- your problem is of the type that is likely to improve after an operation.

This means that surgery is unlikely to be considered as soon as an attack of back pain develops. Other types of treatment will be tried first, and most people recover without the need for an operation.

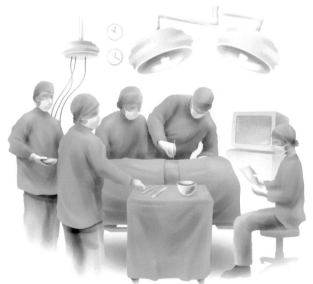

Surgery should be considered only if your symptoms have not responded to other treatment, if you have severe and persisting symptoms, or if your problem is of the type that is likely to improve after an operation.

If you reach the point where an operation is being considered, your surgeon will arrange for detailed investigations to be performed.

Only certain types of back problems are likely to respond well to surgery. In particular there are very good results for those who have severe sciatic pain in the leg. About 80 to 90 per cent of people are very pleased with the results. On the other hand, the success rate is not nearly as good for those whose main problem is pain in the back itself.

What operation?
Removing a disc
There are several different types of back operation. The most common is to remove a prolapsed disc – usually this is the disc between the fourth and fifth lumbar vertebrae or between the fifth lumbar vertebra and the sacrum. In order to prevent any recurrence, the whole disc is usually removed, not just the burst area. Newer techniques include conducting the operation through a small tube and telescope, known as microdiscectomy. This considerably reduces the trauma of the operation so that recovery occurs more rapidly. Some surgeons inject enzymes into the disc or coagulate it electrically, again in an effort to reduce the trauma of the operation.

Bone removal
In some cases the main problem is pressure on the nerve roots from the bone of the vertebral column. The surgeon will aim to relieve this by taking away bone to create more space.

Spinal fusion

Sometimes there is excessive movement between the bones of the vertebral column. The surgeon may decide to fix the vertebrae together. This is known as spinal fusion.

New techniques

Research into surgical procedures inside the disc, including electrical treatments and artificial replacement discs, is currently going on. However, it remains uncertain whether these techniques are worth while.

Convalescence

After surgery you will probably start to get up and walk within a few days. Often you have to wear a lumbar support for a few weeks but you may well get back to light work within a month or two. It will be several months before you can consider doing any heavy manual work. You should always ask your surgeon before undertaking activities that are likely to cause excessive loads on your spine.

Intensive rehabilitation and pain management

A small proportion of people with chronic back pain develop very severe symptoms and become very disabled. There are a number of reasons for this, including not only the mechanical forms of damage around the spine, but also scarring which may develop around the nerve roots. There may be other changes that occur within the central nervous system itself, and the whole problem is often exacerbated by depression, anxiety and fibromyalgia.

Unfortunately, this type of back pain can be very difficult to treat. People in this situation will need a careful and sympathetic assessment, which will include not only analysis of the physical problem but also of their reactions to it.

The next stage is to design an intensive rehabilitation programme tailored to the requirements of each individual, which aims not only to restore physical function but also to help the person concerned to cope with the problem and lead a more normal life.

Important elements of the programme are an understanding of the nature of pain, and that pain does not necessarily mean harm, as well as counselling, learning to pace oneself so that too much is not attempted when feeling a little better, and vocational rehabilitation to enable the person with back pain to return to work.

This type of treatment can be very effective for the most severely disabled back sufferers. Unfortunately the availability of this type of pain management programme is extremely limited and currently is provided at very few centres in Britain. It is hoped that these facilities will become more widely available before too long.

KEY POINTS

- The back pain sufferer should understand how the back works, what goes wrong and why various types of treatment are used

- Exercise is good for the back but sudden forceful movements should be avoided

- The choice of medication is related to the clinical problem. Most patients' pain will be controlled by a simple painkiller such as paracetamol or anti-inflammatory drugs such as ibuprofen

- Surgery is only rarely necessary. On the whole it works a lot better for sciatic pain in the leg than for back pain alone

- Intensive rehabilitation and pain management programmes are effective for people with severe chronic back problems

- The detailed history and the clinical examination form the most important parts of the assessment. Imaging tests are a helpful supplement in appropriate cases

Back pain in young people

Early back pain can persist throughout life

It is a common misconception that back problems are confined to middle-aged and elderly people. It comes as a surprise to realise how common back problems are in children and adolescents. Generally it is a minor discomfort that does not interfere with day-to-day activities, but in some children it may interfere with school work, sport and leisure activities.

About a quarter of all children will have seen their doctor or lost time from school because of backache and, once started in youth, backache frequently persists throughout life.

In most cases investigations show little more than minor wear-and-tear changes, but in a small proportion there may be more significant problems, such as a slipped disc, ankylosing spondylitis (inflammatory form of arthritis – see page 63) or other complaints as described in adults.

The importance of posture and exercise

Poor posture and lack of physical fitness are important but in many young people emotional factors and psychological stress play important roles. Back problems often run in families but whether this is the result of some inherited predisposition, physical factors in family life or emotional responses is commonly difficult to elucidate.

Changes in school life seem to have contributed towards the back problem. Children are now taller than they were a century ago, and yet the average school furniture has remained the same. Hours spent slouching over a desk will aggravate back complaints.

It is important that children do not spend prolonged periods at the desk but get up and walk about and exercise frequently, although for many this does not happen.

As children are of different sizes the desk and chair should be adjustable for height. Ideally the child should be positioned with the back upright, preserving the natural hollow in the low back. The chair seat should slope slightly forward to allow the lumbar spine to curve back slightly. A wedge to tilt the lower body forward slightly may help. The desk should also have a slight slope to make writing easier in the upright position. A poor seating posture will exacerbate back problems.

The same principles will apply to a computer workstation. The screen should be with the upper border at eye level when the child is sitting upright. The chair should be adjustable in height and with a lumbar support.

Another change that has occurred is that children do not use the same desks all the time, but frequently change classrooms. They do not have a desk to call their own. The result is that they have to carry their books with them. Many have a satchel, which can be very heavy, producing strain on the spine and aggravating back symptoms. A rucksack seems a much better way of carrying heavy books, but for many children it is not 'cool'.

We all know that exercise and sports are important and it is generally recognised that children should spend at least two hours a week in physical education,

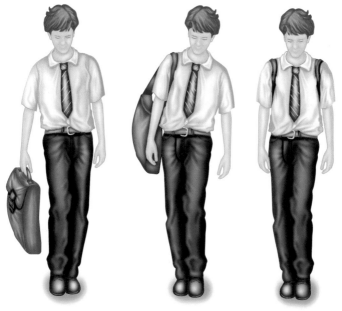

Heavy hand satchels put stress on the spine

Heavy shoulder bags can cause an unnatural spine posture

A well-designed back-pack spreads the load

Back problems are far more common in children than is commonly appreciated. Children often carry heavy bags in one hand or over one shoulder, which can put great stress on the spine.

preferably doing some physical exercise every day. For many, however, this does not happen. Low levels of physical exercise also correlate with the development of back problems.

At the other extreme, children who participate in extreme sports and exercise have an increased risk of injury to the back. These include contact sports, gymnastics, excessive dance and other sporting activities. It is often difficult to achieve the appropriate balance of physical activity.

KEY POINTS

■ Backache in young people is common

■ Commonly, it arises as a result of postural problems and inadequate physical activity

■ Carefully designed desks and chairs will minimise back symptoms

■ Avoid prolonged carrying of heavy bags of books; if this is the case a rucksack is preferable to a satchel or case

■ Undertake regular exercise

Useful addresses

There are several national societies that are concerned with the welfare of people with back pain and with raising funds for research for better methods of diagnosis and treatment. Several of these organisations produce helpful booklets that provide useful factual information.

Arthritis and Musculoskeletal Alliance
Bride House, 18–20 Bride Lane
London EC4Y 8EE
Tel: 020 7842 0910
Fax: 020 7842 0901
Email: arma@rheumatology.org.uk
Website: www.arma.uk.net

UK umbrella association for support groups, professional bodies and research organisations in the field of arthritis and musculoskeletal conditions.

Arthritis Research Campaign
Copeman House, St Mary's Court, St Mary's Gate

Chesterfield S41 7TD
Tel: 01246 558033
Fax: 01246 558007
Helpline: 0870 850 5000
Email: info@arc.org.uk
Website: www.arc.org.uk

Finances an extensive programme of research and education in a wide range of arthritis and rheumatism problems including back pain. Provides useful booklets explaining the various back problems and ways of coping with them.

Arthritis Care
18 Stephenson Way
London NW1 2HD
Tel: 020 7380 6500
Fax: 020 7380 6505
Helplines:
0808 800 4050 (12 noon–4pm Mon–Fri)
020 7380 6555 (10am–4pm)
For those under 26: 0808 808 2000 (10am–2pm Mon–Fri)
Email: helplines@arthritiscare.org.uk
Website: www.arthritiscare.org.uk

Provides information and advice for those who are disabled by all forms of arthritis and back pain. In particular the charity runs holiday hotels for people disabled with arthritis and publishes a bi-monthly newsletter, *Arthritis News*, which is sent to all members. Has network of local branches and support groups.

Back Care
16 Elmtree Road
Teddington TW11 8ST
Tel: 020 8977 5474
Fax: 020 8943 5318
Helpline: 0870 950 0275 (Mon and Fri 9am–12 noon;
Wed 6–9pm)
Email: info@backcare.org.uk
Website: www.backcare.org.uk

Has local branches throughout the country with
regular meetings to disseminate information and
advice for people with back pain. Its mission is to fund
patient-oriented scientific research into the causes and
treatment of back pain, to educate people to use their
bodies sensibly and so reduce the incidence of back
pain, and to form and support branches through
which sufferers and those who care for them may
receive information, advice and mutual help.

Benefits Enquiry Line
Helpline: 0800 882200
Minicom: 0800 243355
Website: www.dwp.gov.uk
N. Ireland: 0800 220674

Government agency giving information and advice on
sickness and disability benefits for people with
disabilities and their carers.

British Acupuncture Council
63 Jeddo Road
London W12 9HQ
Tel: 020 8735 0400

Fax: 020 8735 0404
Email: info@acupuncture.org.uk
Website: www.acupuncture.org.uk

Professional body representing acupuncturists who have extensive training in acupuncture and biomedical sciences appropriate for the practice of this therapy. Offers lists of qualified acupuncture therapists and can recommend accredited training courses.

British Pain Society
21 Portland Place
London W1B 1PY
Tel: 020 7631 8870
Fax: 020 7323 2015
Email: info@britishpainsociety.org
Website: www.britishpainsociety.org

British chapter of the International Association for the Study of Pain. Multidisciplinary professionals liaising in pain management. Publications available free to members, on the website or for sale.

Chartered Society of Physiotherapy
14 Bedford Row
London WC1R 4ED
Tel: 020 7306 6666
Fax: 020 7306 6611
Email: csp@cphysio.org.uk
Website: www.csp.org.uk

For information about all aspects of physiotherapy. Offers lists of registered physiotherapists around the country.

General Chiropractic Council
44 Wicklow Street
London WC1X 9HL
Tel: 020 7713 5155
Fax: 020 7713 5844
Email: enquiries@gcc-uk.org
Website: www.gcc-uk.org

Professional body for chiropractors which can provide details of registered practitioners in your area.

General Osteopathic Council
176 Tower Bridge Road
London SE1 3LU
Tel: 020 7357 6655
Fax: 020 7357 0011
Email: info@osteopathy.org.uk
Website: www.osteopathy.org.uk

Regulatory body offering information to the public and lists of accredited osteopaths around the country.

National Ankylosing Spondylitis Society
PO Box 179
Mayfield, East Sussex TN20 6ZL
Tel: 01435 873527
Fax: 01435 873027
Email: nass@nass.co.uk
Website: www.nass.co.uk

For patients with ankylosing spondylitis, their families and friends, and doctors and research workers concerned with this problem. Provides practical advice and help, and holds open meetings for members. Has over 100 branches providing supervised physiotherapy one evening a week. Video, cassette tapes and CD-ROM of physiotherapy exercise available as well as guidebook, a twice-yearly journal and other publications.

National Institute for Health and Clinical Excellence (NICE)

MidCity Place, 71 High Holborn
London WC1V 6NA
Tel: 020 7067 5800
Fax: 020 7067 5801
Email: nice@nice.nhs.uk
Website: www.nice.org.uk

Provides national guidance on the promotion of good health and the prevention and treatment of ill-health. Patient information leaflets are available for each piece of guidance issued.

National Osteoporosis Society

Camerton
Bath BA2 0PJ
Tel: 01761 471771
Fax: 01761 471104
Helpline: 0845 450 0230
Email: info@nos.org.uk
Website: www.nos.org.uk

A charitable organisation providing advice and support for people with osteoporosis and seeking to improve general awareness and to sponsor research into this problem. Helpline staffed by specially trained nurses. Has local support groups.

Prodigy Website
Sowerby Centre for Health Informatics at Newcastle
(SCHIN), Bede House, All Saints Business Centre
Newcastle upon Tyne NE1 2ES
Tel: 0191 243 6100
Fax: 0191 243 6101
Email: prodigy-enquiries@schin.co.uk
Website: www.prodigy.nhs.uk/PILS/indexself.asp

A website mainly for GPs giving information for
patients listed by disease plus named self-help
organisations.

Spinal Injuries Association
2 Trueman Place, Oldbrook
Milton Keynes MK6 2HH
Tel: 0845 678 6633
Fax: 0845 070 6911
Helpline: 0800 980 0501 (Mon–Fri 9.30am–1pm and
2–4.30pm)
Email: sia@spinal.co.uk
Website: www.spinal.co.uk

For people with spinal cord injury, their families and
friends. Offers a range of services for paraplegics and
tetraplegics. Publishes a regular newsletter with useful
practical advice and help.

The internet as a source of further information

After reading this book, you may feel that you would
like further information on the subject. The internet is

of course an excellent place to look and there are many websites with useful information about medical disorders, related charities and support groups.

It should always be remembered, however, that the internet is unregulated and anyone is free to set up a website and add information to it. Many websites offer impartial advice and information that has been compiled and checked by qualified medical professionals. Some, on the other hand, are run by commercial organisations with the purpose of promoting their own products. Others still are run by pressure groups, some of which will provide carefully assessed and accurate information whereas others may be suggesting medications or treatments that are not supported by the medical and scientific community.

Unless you know the address of the website you want to visit – for example, www.familydoctor.co.uk – you may find the following guidelines useful when searching the internet for information.

Search engines and other searchable sites

Google (www.google.co.uk) is the most popular search engine used in the UK, followed by Yahoo! (http://uk.yahoo.com) and MSN (www.msn.co.uk). Also popular are the search engines provided by Internet Service Providers such as Tiscali and other sites such as the BBC site (www.bbc.co.uk).

In addition to the search engines that index the whole web, there are also medical sites with search facilities, which act almost like mini-search engines, but cover only medical topics or even a particular area of medicine. Again, it is wise to look at who is responsible for compiling the information offered to ensure that it is impartial and medically accurate. The NHS Direct site (www.nhsdirect.nhs.uk) is an example of a searchable medical site.

Links to many British medical charities can be found at the Association of Medical Research Charities' website (www.amrc.org.uk) and at Charity Choice (www.charitychoice.co.uk).

Search phrases

Be specific when entering a search phrase. Searching for information on 'cancer' will return results for many different types of cancer as well as on cancer in general. You may even find sites offering astrological information. More useful results will be returned by using search phrases such as 'lung cancer' and 'treatments for lung cancer'. Both Google and Yahoo! offer an advanced search option that includes the ability to search for the exact phrase; enclosing the search phrase in quotes, that is, 'treatments for lung cancer', will have the same effect. Limiting a search to an exact phrase reduces the number of results returned but it is best to refine a search to an exact match only if you are not getting useful results with a normal search. Adding 'UK' to your search term will bring up mainly British sites, so a good phrase might be 'lung cancer' UK (don't include UK within the quotes).

Always remember the internet is international and unregulated. It holds a wealth of valuable information but individual sites may be biased, out of date or just plain wrong. Family Doctor Publications accepts no responsibility for the content of links published in this series.

Index

Your pages

We have included the following pages because they may help you manage your illness or condition and its treatment.

Before an appointment with a health professional, it can be useful to write down a short list of questions of things that you do not understand, so that you can make sure that you do not forget anything.

Some of the sections may not be relevant to your circumstances.

We are always pleased to receive constructive criticism or suggestions about how to improve the books. You can contact us at:

Email: familydoctor@btinternet.com
Letter: Family Doctor Publications
         PO Box 4664
         Poole
         BH15 1NN

Thank you

Health-care contact details

Name:

Job title:

Place of work:

Tel:

Name:

Job title:

Place of work:

Tel:

Name:

Job title:

Place of work:

Tel:

Name:

Job title:

Place of work:

Tel:

Significant past health events – illnesses/ operations/investigations/treatments

Event	Month	Year	Age (at time)

Appointments for health care

Name:

Place:

Date:

Time:

Tel:

Name:

Place:

Date:

Time:

Tel:

Name:

Place:

Date:

Time:

Tel:

Name:

Place:

Date:

Time:

Tel:

Appointments for health care

Name:

Place:

Date:

Time:

Tel:

Name:

Place:

Date:

Time:

Tel:

Name:

Place:

Date:

Time:

Tel:

Name:

Place:

Date:

Time:

Tel:

Current medication(s) prescribed by your doctor

Medicine name:

Purpose:

Frequency & dose:

Start date:

End date:

Medicine name:

Purpose:

Frequency & dose:

Start date:

End date:

Medicine name:

Purpose:

Frequency & dose:

Start date:

End date:

Medicine name:

Purpose:

Frequency & dose:

Start date:

End date:

Other medicines/supplements you are taking, not prescribed by your doctor

Medicine/treatment:

Purpose:

Frequency & dose:

Start date:

End date:

Medicine/treatment:

Purpose:

Frequency & dose:

Start date:

End date:

Medicine/treatment:

Purpose:

Frequency & dose:

Start date:

End date:

Medicine/treatment:

Purpose:

Frequency & dose:

Start date:

End date:

Questions to ask at appointments
(Note: do bear in mind that doctors work under great time pressure, so long lists may not be helpful for either of you)

Questions to ask at appointments
(Note: do bear in mind that doctors work under great time pressure, so long lists may not be helpful for either of you)

Notes